The Nurses' Career Guide Companion Workbook

The
Nurses'
Career Guide

Companion Workbook

Zardoya E. Eagles, R.N.

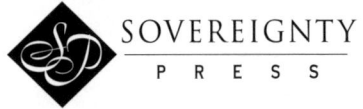

SOVEREIGNTY
P R E S S

The Nurses' Career Guide Companion Workbook
© 1997 by Zardoya E. Eagles

Sovereignty Press
1241 Johnson Avenue, #353
San Luis Obispo, CA   93401

Manufactured in the United States of America
First printing October 1997
04 03 02 01 00 99 98 97   10 9 8 7 6 5 4 3 2 1

Cover illustration by Jorel Williams, Minneapolis, Minnesota
Cover design © 1997 by Lightbourne Images, Ashland, Oregon
Editing by Mark Wilson, San Rafael, California
Interior design by Zardoya Eagles, San Luis Obispo, California

ISBN 0-9656025-0-8

. . . .

*If one advances confidently in the direction of his dreams,
and endeavors to live the life which he has imagined,
he will meet with success unexpected in common hours.*

– Thoreau

Contents

Introduction

This workbook is designed to be used in conjunction with *The Nurses' Career Guide: Discovering New Horizons in Health Care* written by Zardoya Eagles, R.N. Its convenient format allows you to:

- keep all of your responses in one place as you work through the exercises found in *The Nurses' Career Guide*

- use the page numbers at the beginning of each section to easily refer to the corresponding section of the book

- further expand on your own thoughts and ideas in the blank pages left for you

Let the writing begin!

People can be divided into three groups:
those who make things happen,
those who watch things happen,
and those who wonder what happened.

— John W. Newbern

Current Changes in Health Care

Problem or Opportunity?

*If you want to truly understand something,
try to change it.*

— Kurt Lewin

YOUR PROFESSIONAL JOURNEY (pp. 7–23)

Briefly describe your "professional journey" as a nurse. Why did you decide to go into nursing? How did you select your area of expertise? Do you remember your vision for the future when you entered this profession? Has that vision changed? How have you dealt with the changes you've encountered in your work environment?

. . . .

Assessment

Whether you think you can or think you can't, you're right.

— Henry Ford

UNIVERSAL JOB SKILLS (pp. 29–30)

Take a moment to look at these eight "universal" job skills. How do each of these skills play a role in your work as a nurse?

1. Leadership/persuasion

2. Problem-solving/creativity

3. Working as part of a team

4. Manual dexterity

5. Helping/instructing others

6. Initiative

7. Frequent public contact

8. Physical stamina

EXERCISE 1: YOUR REACTIONS TO CHANGE (pp. 31–33)

Take some time to reflect on the changes you have faced in the past few years and how you have reacted to them. Identify the changes that have occurred in your workplace in the past few years. Identify how your peers reacted, and try to identify the agents of change in your workplace.

How about those in your personal life?

Write them on the following table:

Changes I have gone through in the past few years	How did I react personally?	What were the advantages and disadvantages?

Changes I have gone through in the past few years	How did I react personally?	What were the advantages and disadvantages?

Changes I have gone through in the past few years	How did I react personally?	What were the advantages and disadvantages?

As you examine your responses to change, identify how resistance to change manifests in your behavior.

What, if anything, would you have done differently?

What are some of the effective ways that you have dealt with change?

What are some of the ineffective ways that you have dealt with change?

Is there any one type of change (in the workplace or in your personal life) that is hardest for you to deal with?

Identify three areas you would like to work on to find more creative and self-affirming ways of adapting to change. You may want to write them as if you were writing short-term/long-term goals for your patients.

EXERCISE 2: VALUES CLARIFICATION (pp.33–36)

Set aside some time in which you can be alone, quiet, and introspective. You can just write down ideas as they come to you, or you can use the following suggestions as a guide.

Here is a list of commonly stated values that you can use to trigger your process, if you choose:

Physical health	Spirituality/Religion
Education	Intellectual development
Mental health	Justice/Truth
Family/Friends	Community involvement
Financial security	Fulfilling career

Evaluate the highest priorities in your life. Which are the most important to you? List 5 to 10, or even more.

Now prioritize your values, placing them in order from most to least important.

Use the following form to describe ideal behaviors that would fit within the framework of each value. Ask yourself: "If I were living that value perfectly, what would my behavior be like?" Then, write value statements for each of these prioritized values.

Value:

Ideal behaviors:

Value statement:

Value:

Ideal behaviors:

Value statement:

Value:
Ideal behaviors:
Value statement:
Value:
Ideal behaviors:
Value statement:

Value:

Ideal behaviors:

Value statement:

Value:

Ideal behaviors:

Value statement:

EXERCISE 3: WORK HISTORY (pp. 36–37)

Complete the form on pages 24 and 25. Note that "work experience" can mean community and/or volunteer activities in addition to past employment. Then, come back and answer the following questions:

1) What was your favorite work experience? Why?

2) What was you least favorite work experience? Why?

3) What was your most significant contribution? Why?

4) What was your favorite activity on your most recent job?

5) What did you find challenging or stimulating about your most recent job?

6) Go through the work history form on pages 24 and 25, and compile a list of the skills or "action words" you used to describe what you most enjoyed and what you consider to be your greatest achievements.

Work experience and dates	Title or job description	What I enjoyed most	What I enjoyed least	My most significant achievement or contribution

Work experience and dates	Title or job description	What I enjoyed most	What I enjoyed least	My most significant achievement or contribution

EXERCISE 4: FAVORITE ACTIVITIES (pp. 38–43)

Examine the list of words on pages 38–42 in *The Nurses' Career Guide*. As you examine this list, focus not only on your professional life, but on your personal life as well. Look at any roles you play: in the family, at work, in the community, at church, etc. Write down any skills or activities that you regularly perform and have found the most *enjoyable, fulfilling, and rewarding*. You may want to assign your most favorite activities a special mark.

Can you identify any patterns or similarities among the words on your list?

Do you perform the activities you selected in your current job, or are they totally different from what you are now doing?

Now, select your top five skills—those five activities that really make you feel alive, engaged, and happy when you are doing them.

Rank these five in order of priority, with the one you most enjoy first.

Use the following form to write down at least two examples from your experience that describe your greatest achievement while performing each of these activities. What did you do? How did you do it? What was the result?

Prioritized skill:

Examples:
1)

2)

Prioritized skill:

Examples:
1)

2)

Prioritized skill:

Examples:
1)

2)

Prioritized skill:

Examples:
1)

2)

Prioritized skill:

Examples:
1)

2)

EXERCISE 5: PERSONAL ACHIEVEMENTS (pp.43–45)

Make a list of your personal achievements. For each achievement, identify the predominant activity or activities that were involved in your success.

Examine this list of achievements, skills, and activities for *patterns*, and note any similarities you identify. Correlate the skills and activities related to your achievements listed above with the activities you identified as most enjoyable, fulfilling, and rewarding in Exercises 3 and 4 by filling in the form on page 34.

Are there any similarities or patterns that emerge?

Are you utilizing the parts of yourself that you most value in your current job? Or maybe in another part of your life, like the PTA or your church?

How much of your day is spent doing things you really enjoy? Where are the gaps between what you *love to do* and what you *really do*?

Are there any ways to integrate the two, so that you are doing what you love?

EXERCISE 6: WANT ADS (pp.46–47)

Go through the want ads in the Sunday paper, *The Wall Street Journal*, nursing magazines, job guides, online web sites, or other sources of employment advertisement, and carefully read the ads for what skills they require of an applicant. In the space below, write down any aspects of these descriptions that you know you *can* and *want* to do. Do this for at least ten different ads, and *don't just focus on nursing jobs—read them all!* It does not matter if you qualify for the job or not, because what you want to identify here are *skills* and ideas for types of work you could enjoy.

Now, as you scan your list, choose your top ten skills and rank them in order with your favorite first.

Compare this list with those you compiled for Exercises 3, 4, and 5 by completing the following form:

Exercise 3 Past work experiences	Exercise 4 Favorite skills and activities	Exercise 5 Greatest achievements	Exercise 6 Want ads job description

Do you notice any similarities?

If you have any skills or activities that show up on more than one list, just cross them off. From the remaining skills and activities, select your top five favorite activities, and rank them in order of priority.

Master Skills and Activities List
1.
2.
3.
4.
5.

EXERCISE 7: IDEAL JOB/BUSINESS (pp. 47–48)

1) Describe your ideal job.

2) What, if anything, do you think could stop you from being able to have this job? Why?

3) If you identified a "stopper" in the above question, describe what you would have to do to get past the obstacles and clear the pathway for you to have what you want in the workplace. Be specific.

4) If you could start your own business, what would it be?

5) What, if anything, do you think could stop you from being able to start this business? Why?

6) If you identified a "stopper" in the above question, go back to your ideal world and describe what you would have to do to get past these obstacles and clear the pathway for you to be able to develop the type of business you want. Be specific.

Planning

*Every great personal victory was preceded by a personal
goal or dream—a dream that sprang from
the value core of some individual.*

— Dennis R. Webb

CAREER OPPORTUNITIES (pp. 53–84)

Use your Master Skills and Activities List as you read through the career options in chapter 4 of *The Nurses' Career Guide*. If any of the options interest you, see if you can find a match between the skills required for that job and the skills you've listed as the ones you most enjoy. Write down any of your skills that may apply next to the career options listed below:

Inpatient career options for nurses

Hospital-based nursing

Nurse manager

Education and training

Utilization review

Discharge planning

Case management

Risk management

Outpatient career options for nurses

Home care

Long-term care

Cardiac rehabilitation

Rehabilitation nursing

Outpatient clinics

Outpatient surgical centers

Community education

Community nursing centers

Community nursing organizations

Forensic nursing and sexual assault nurse examiners

Non-patient care and business career options for nurses

Quality assurance

Utilization review

Case management

Occupational health

Workers' compensation

Telephone triage and advice lines

Sales

In-Service education and training

Nurse consulting

Medical-legal nurse consultant

Nursing instructor

Entrepreneurship

MENTORSHIP (pp. 85–97)

Is mentorship right for you?

First, identify what (not *who*) you need. Make a list of the kinds of help you'd like to have. Ask yourself, "If I were as successful as I wanted to be right now, what would be happening?"

Next, evaluate yourself as a prospective mentee. Are you resistant to receiving help from others? What are your reasons?

How do you really feel about becoming a mentee?

How dependent are you willing to become?

How can you maintain a balance between dependence and independence?

Are you willing or able to ask someone for help?

Is it difficult for you to be in the passive, receiving role instead of the giving role?

Selecting a mentor

Now, identify some mentor candidates. Go through your list of needs above, and make a list of possible mentors. Who do you know that thinks you have potential? Who has recently achieved what you want and might be inspired by this new success to help you? Who has helped you in the past and might help again?

As you look at your completed list, ask yourself some questions about each candidate:

Where are the potential mentors in terms of their own careers?

Are they just beginning, or are they perhaps switching career fields?

How influential are they?

Do they hold any office, or have they received any honors?

What is their current situation?

Have these potential mentors ever helped others? In what ways?

How do they feel about mentoring?

Can you talk to their former protégés?

If you already know potential mentors, evaluate your relationship with them. Would adding the mentor-mentee dimension have a positive or negative effect?

Do you share similar goals and values with these people?

If they are very different from you but can be of great help, try to identify ways to work around (or at least tolerate) the differences for as long as the relationship is valuable.

Contacting your mentor

Do you have any mutual acquaintances who could recommend you to a potential mentor that you do not know?

If you do not have a personal contact, write the person a letter. Try to compliment the person on something she has done, and share something about yourself that will spark some interest. If you can think of something that you could do for her, by all means, mention it. If it pertains to a project, include examples of your work, if possible.

Doing your homework

Be sure to do your homework before you meet your potential mentor. Decide on your personal agenda and what you want the meeting's outcome to be. Record that below. Be sure you are clear about your needs, your goals, and your vision.

Goals (pp. 99–106)

Complete the following statement, listing every idea that comes into your mind:

"Someday I'm going to . . ."

Your Personal Action Plan

The following form, your Personal Action Plan, can be used to direct your activities as you work to achieve your goals. First, refer to your core values, which you identified in Exercise 2 in Section 2 of this workbook. Write your value statement at the top of the page, followed by your long-term goal. Use as many pages as you need; each long term-goal gets a page.

Once you have written out your long-term goals, determine what major steps you would have to undertake to accomplish each goal. Record these short-term goals on the form under your long-term goal.

Now, break it down even further into the actual *tasks* that need to be completed. This list should include anything, no matter how small, that needs to be accomplished to reach your goals. Record any time deadlines that apply, and check off tasks as they are completed.

When you plan your month, or your week, or your day, you can refer to these pages to determine what needs to be done—and by when—for you to achieve your goal.

Personal Action Plan

Value:

Long-Term Goal:

Short-Term Goals:

X	Tasks	Deadline

Personal Action Plan

Value:

Long-Term Goal:

Short-Term Goals:

X	Tasks	Deadline

Personal Action Plan

Value:

Long-Term Goal:

Short-Term Goals:

X	Tasks	Deadline

Personal Action Plan

Value:

Long-Term Goal:

Short-Term Goals:

X	Tasks	Deadline

Personal Action Plan

Value:

Long-Term Goal:

Short-Term Goals:

X	Tasks	Deadline

Personal Action Plan

Value:

Long-Term Goal:

Short-Term Goals:

X	Tasks	Deadline

Personal Action Plan

Value:

Long-Term Goal:

Short-Term Goals:

X	Tasks	Deadline

Implementation

*Things which matter most
must never be at the mercy of things which matter least.*

— Goethe

RÉSUMÉS (pp. 112–123)

Planning your résumé

A good place to start is to organize your data—sift through your past achievements, work history, experiences, education, and all the other information covered in Sections 2 and 3, and fill in the following data sheet:

RÉSUMÉ DATA SHEET

Name:

Address:

Phone: (   )

Fax: (   )

E-mail:

Education (list school, city/state, and degree or major):

1.

2.

3.

States licensed in:

Certifications:

Professional memberships:

1.

2.

3.

Publications (list article and name of publication):

1.

2.

3.

Presentations:

1.

2.

3.

Committees/Special projects:

Employment History

Month/Year (from-to)	Job Title	Employer	City/State

Description of responsibilities (action-based, 2 or 3 sentences):

Month/Year (from-to)	Job Title	Employer	City/State

Description of responsibilities (action-based, 2 or 3 sentences):

Employment History

Month/Year (from-to)	Job Title	Employer	City/State

Description of responsibilities (action-based, 2 or 3 sentences):

Month/Year (from-to)	Job Title	Employer	City/State

Description of responsibilities (action-based, 2 or 3 sentences):

Employment History

Month/Year (from-to)	Job Title	Employer	City/State

Description of responsibilities (action-based, 2 or 3 sentences):

Month/Year (from-to)	Job Title	Employer	City/State

Description of responsibilities (action-based, 2 or 3 sentences):

Employment History

Month/Year (from–to)	Job Title	Employer	City/State

Description of responsibilities (action–based, 2 or 3 sentences):

Month/Year (from–to)	Job Title	Employer	City/State

Description of responsibilities (action–based, 2 or 3 sentences):

Go through your Employment History Sheets and highlight any action words. These words will be used in your résumé to start each sentence with an action word. Create your own personal list of action words below.

Writing your résumé

Now, using the sample résumés from the Resources Guide in the back of *The Nurses' Career Guide,* create your own résumé or résumés. Do your rough draft below using the guidelines on pages 116–122. Then, following the tips on page 123, have your résumé typed or typeset on a computer to create the finished document.

INFORMATIONAL INTERVIEWING (pp. 124–140)

List of contacts

Using the information from Chapter 4 on career options, determine at least three options you would consider as possibilities for meeting your goals. Write each of the three on a separate page and, underneath them, write down names of people you know who work in that area. If you don't know of any people, begin by making a list of places and/or people you could contact who might be able to recommend someone for you to interview.

Letter of approach

This letter should: 1) introduce yourself, 2) explain why you are contacting them, 3) outline what you hope to accomplish by meeting with them, and 4) advise them that you will follow up by phone. Remember to make your expectations clear by including a statement such as: "Please understand that I do not expect you to know of or have any positions at this time. I would, however, greatly appreciate your advice and insight about _____."

Setting the appointment

Write out a script for your follow-up call below:

"Two-minute drill"

Write out the introduction for your two-minute drill (also known as your "change of shift report") below, following the guidelines on pages 136–137 of *The Nurses' Career Guide.*

Sample questions

Here are some sample informational interview questions for you to use or to help build your own list:

How did you get into this work?

What do you like most about it?

What do you like least about it?

What is your typical day like?

What are your biggest frustrations with this work?

What are your biggest rewards?

What type of academic and/or work background is generally required to enter this field?

Do you belong to any professional organizations or alliances?

How important is it to join?

Is this a growing field?

What potential exists for advancement?

If you were starting out again, what would you do differently?

What companies do you know of that hire people to do this type of work?

How would you suggest I proceed in seeking a job in this field?

What is the range of salary for entry-level positions?

What income level should I expect to reach with my background and qualifications?

What types of reorganization and/or restructuring has this industry experienced?

What were the results?

Are there any indications or plans for future reorganization or restructuring?

What specific areas do you feel promise the most growth?

If you were to leave your kind of work, what other kind of work would attract you?

If you were hiring someone right now, what would be the most critical factors determining your selection?

Thank-you letter

Write a rough draft thank-you letter or note below.

Follow-up

It is actually easy to keep track of all this information if you just use the simple form on the following page.

INFORMATIONAL INTERVIEWING DATA SHEET

Name/Title/Company Address	Phone number	Date letter sent	Date of interview
	Referred by	Date of phone contact	Date thank-you sent
Pertinent Information/Advice:		Planned follow-through	
		Names of referrals received	
Name/Title/Company Address	Phone number	Date letter sent	Date of interview
	Referred by	Date of phone contact	Date thank-you sent
Pertinent Information/Advice:		Planned follow-through	
		Names of referrals received	

INFORMATIONAL INTERVIEWING DATA SHEET

Name/Title/Company Address	Phone number	Date letter sent	Date of interview
	Referred by	Date of phone contact	Date thank-you sent
Pertinent Information/Advice:		Planned follow-through	
		Names of referrals received	
Name/Title/Company Address	Phone number	Date letter sent	Date of interview
	Referred by	Date of phone contact	Date thank-you sent
Pertinent Information/Advice:		Planned follow-through	
		Names of referrals received	

INFORMATIONAL INTERVIEWING DATA SHEET

Name/Title/Company Address	Phone number	Date letter sent	Date of interview
	Referred by	Date of phone contact	Date thank-you sent
Pertinent Information/Advice:		Planned follow-through	
		Names of referrals received	
Name/Title/Company Address	Phone number	Date letter sent	Date of interview
	Referred by	Date of phone contact	Date thank-you sent
Pertinent Information/Advice:		Planned follow-through	
		Names of referrals received	

INFORMATIONAL INTERVIEWING DATA SHEET

Name/Title/Company Address	Phone number	Date letter sent	Date of interview
	Referred by	Date of phone contact	Date thank-you sent
Pertinent Information/Advice:		Planned follow-through	
		Names of referrals received	
Name/Title/Company Address	Phone number	Date letter sent	Date of interview
	Referred by	Date of phone contact	Date thank-you sent
Pertinent Information/Advice:		Planned follow-through	
		Names of referrals received	

INFORMATIONAL INTERVIEWING DATA SHEET

Name/Title/Company Address	Phone number	Date letter sent	Date of interview
	Referred by	Date of phone contact	Date thank-you sent
Pertinent Information/Advice:		Planned follow-through	
		Names of referrals received	
Name/Title/Company Address	Phone number	Date letter sent	Date of interview
	Referred by	Date of phone contact	Date thank-you sent
Pertinent Information/Advice:		Planned follow-through	
		Names of referrals received	

COVER LETTERS (pp. 140–143)

Following the guidelines on pages 141–142, create your rough draft cover letter below:

JOB INTERVIEWING (pp. 143–149)

Vital information

For each of the companies you are planning to interview with, record vital information below. Use the guidelines on pages 143–144 of *The Nurses' Career Guide* to give you ideas as to what to look for.

Your bottom line

What are you willing to accept in terms of hours, working conditions, salary, and other provisions of employment?

Use the following form to record your monthly spending plan:

Expense	Monthly Itemized	Monthly Total
Groceries: Food		
Household supplies		
School lunches		Groceries:
Home: Mortgage or Rent		
Homeowner' or Renter's Ins.		Home:
Utilities: Electricity		
Gas		
Water		
Phone		
Garbage		
Other		Utilities:
Clothing:		
Dry cleaning and laundry		Clothing:

Expense	Monthly Itemized	Monthly Total
Auto: Car payment		
Gasoline and oil		
Repair		
Auto insurance		Auto:
Household: Yard expenses		
Repairs, improvements, maintainance		
Domestic help		
Other		Household:
Recreation/Entertainment: Sports		
Weekend entertainment (movies, dining out)		
Club dues (country club, fitness)		
Babysitter		
Other		Recreation:

Expense	Monthly Itemized	Monthly Total
Family: Adult (classes, piano lessons, etc.)		
Children/Daycare		**Family:**
Gifts: Birthdays (family, friends, relatives)		
Weddings		
Mother's/Father's Day		
Christmas/Hannukah fund		
Other		**Gifts:**
Publications: Books		
Magazines		
Newspapers		**Publications:**
Medical: Doctors/Chiropractors		
Dentists		
Drugs/Medications		**Medical:**

Expense	Monthly Itemized	Monthly Total
Miscellaneous/Slush Fund:		Misc:
Contributions:		Contrib:
Other:		Other:
Monthly Expenses Total: (add together all categories)		
x 12		
Annual Total:		

Filling in this form gives you two vital pieces of information:

1. Your monthly expenses/income requirement.

2. Your annual income bottom line.

Use these numbers as a guideline when you make a decision about a job and/or salary offer. Your bottom line is just as important as any corporate bottom line!

Break down your hourly or monthly income to the number of hours you *really* work—commute time and preparation time included—to get a clearer picture of what you earn. Use the form below:

1) Wages ($ per hour):	
2) Hours worked per day:	
3) Total $ per day:	
4) Extra time: Commute:	
Preparation:	
Miscellaneous:	
5) Total extra time:	
6) Total hours put into job (#2 + #5):	
True hourly wage (#3 ÷ #6):	

What is the highest salary you would hope to earn?

What is the absolute lowest amount, under which you simply cannot afford to go?

What is the standard salary range for the position you are interviewing for?

Preparation (pp. 144–147)

Be certain you can answer the following key questions:

1) "Why did you pick *our* organization instead of seeking a job somewhere else?"

2) "What are your skills and achievements, and do they match our needs?"

3) "What kind of person are you?"

4) "What sets you apart from all the other people who can do the same thing?"

5) "Can we afford you?"

Be prepared to find the answers to the following questions:

1) What does this job require?

2) Are my skills a "good match" for this job?

3) Are these the kind of people I enjoy working with?

4) What sets me apart from all the others who can also do this job, and how can I convey this to you?

5) Can I persuade you to hire me and pay me the salary I want?

Thank-you letter

Below, create a draft thank-you letter to an interviewer, using the guidelines on pages 149–150 in *The Nurses' Career Guide.*

Evaluation

*What lies behind us and what lies before us
are tiny matters
compared to what lies within us.*

— Oliver Wendell Holmes

SUCCESS (pp. 157–167)

Contemplate your perceptions of success. How much of a role have Grand Goals played in your life, your decisions, and your relationships?

You may want to return to Sections 2 and 3 to review the results of the exercises you did there. First, look at your values clarification from Section 2. Do you find any pitfalls or mind-traps among them? Or are they in alignment with your big-picture view of your life?

New Insights

Carefully examine the goals you wrote in Section 3. Note any new insights you may have gained since you initially wrote them.